GASTRIC SLEEVE COOKBOOK:

**FLUID and PUREE –
30+ Shakes, Drinks, Broth and Puree
recipes for early stages of post-weight
loss surgery diet**

Selena Lancaster

Disclaimer

The information contained in this eBook does not constitute
medical advice. Readers who are in need of medical advice
should consult a physician and/or a medical health professional.
Readers who are in need of specific dietary advice relating to
their condition should consult a dietician and/or a medical
health professional.

If you think you are suffering from a medical condition, you
should seek professional health services right away. Do not
delay seeking medical advice, or forego medical advice already
given, because of any information presented in this eBook .

No warranties are given in relation to the medical information
presented in this eBook. No liability will accrue to the writer
and/or eBook publisher in the event that the reader and/or user
suffers any loss as a result of reliance, in part or in full, upon the
information presented in this eBook.

Get a BONUS gift exclusive to my readers for FREE!

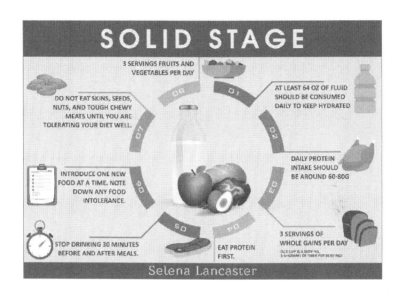

- *A4-sized printable **Complete Food List Poster** for fluid and puree stages*
- *A4-sized printable Daily **Dietary Reminders Posters** for all post-surgery stages*

Scan the QR code and get yours now!

FLUID AND PUREE

GASTRIC SLEEVE COOKBOOK

CONTENT

Part I Introduction

The battle against obesity has become a worldwide effort. According to the World Health Organization's data in 2014, more than 1.9 billion adults worldwide were considered overweight. Of this number, around 600 million individuals were considered as obese. In addition, around 41 million children under the age of 5 were obese or overweight as of 2014.

In the media, non-profit groups and charitable organizations raise awareness on the plight of undernourished populations in areas suffering from severe drought, natural calamities, civil or political unrest, war, and other natural or man-made disasters. Humanitarian efforts to stave off malnutrition are worthy causes to be supported, but it is striking to know that the majority of the world's population lives in countries where obesity, rather than malnutrition, kills more individuals each year.

Classifying adults as either overweight or obese requires an analysis of their body mass index (BMI). By definition, BMI refers to the person's weight in kilograms divided by the square of his height in meters (kg/m2). The WHO defines an adult as overweight if his/her BMI is equal to or greater than 25. If the adult individual's BMI is equal to or greater than 30, he or she is considered obese. The standards of overweight and obese for children under 5 and those between 5-19 years of age vary slightly from the standard for adults.

Obesity is a major health concern globally because of the myriad of illnesses and medical conditions linked directly or indirectly to it. Some of the medical conditions and diseases that are caused by obesity include high blood pressure, high cholesterol, stroke, heart disease, diabetes, certain cancers (i.e. kidney, colon, breast, and esophagus), osteoarthritis, gout, gallbladder disease, gallstones, sleep apnea, asthma, and many more.

Physicians and health experts have always raised awareness and preached the importance of an overall healthy lifestyle to battle overweight and obesity, including proper nutrition, regular exercise, proper amounts of sleep, and other positive lifestyle choices. Sadly, however, for so many people it really is a daunting challenge to try to reverse what may be years of poor nutrition and habits, and weight loss can be an extremely difficult goal.

Weight-loss surgeries

For individuals who have a body mass index (BMI) of 40 or higher, or about 100 pounds overweight for adult men and about 80 pounds overweight for adult women, one option that doctors may offer is weight loss surgery, especially if other options for weight loss such as diet plans and exercise routines have not succeeded significantly.

Weight loss surgery may also be recommended for obese individuals who have not reached the 40 BMI level yet, but are at serious risk of conditions such as type 2 diabetes, high cholesterol, heart disease, or severe sleep apnea. For individuals considering weight loss surgery, all risks are also discussed in detail, as well as lifestyle changes that need to be followed in accordance with the requirements before and after the weight loss surgery.

Dr. Linda Zhang, an assistant professor of surgery at Mount Sinai Hospital, explained to the *New York Daily News* in an interview that weight loss surgeries are not just about aesthetics or looking better. "This is about your overall health and life expectancy," she said. "Having obesity causes a lot of other medical problems: diabetes, high blood pressure, high cholesterol, obstructive sleep apnea, heart disease, arthritis and asthma. One of the great things about bariatric surgeries is that they both help people lose weight and dramatically improve all of these co-related medical problems."

Weight loss surgeries are classified into broad groups: restrictive, malabsorptive, and through electrical device implants. Restrictive surgeries are designed to shrink the stomach size so the patient can eat less food, promoting weight loss. A popular restrictive weight loss surgery is gastric banding, which squeezes the stomach into an upper and lower section with the use of an inflatable band.

Malabsorptive surgeries not only reduce the stomach size but also the digestive tract so the body absorbs less calories. Also known as intestinal bypasses, malabsorptive surgeries are rarely performed on their own these days (usually, in conjunction with restrictive surgeries) because of side effects. The most popular type of weight loss surgery, the gastric bypass surgery (also called Roux-En-Y Gastric Bypass), is a combination of restrictive and malabsorptive weight loss surgeries.

A newer method being used is the Maestro Rechargeable System, which utilizes an electrical device implanted in the abdomen. This devices sends electrical signals to the vagus nerve, a nerve connecting the stomach to the brain, indicating when the stomach is full. A remote control is used for this device, and can be programmed to turn on or off at certain periods, telling the brain that the stomach can no longer take in food.

Side effects

Weight loss surgical procedures do have side effects which vary from patient to patient. For gastric banding, for instance, common risks include vomiting after ingesting too much food at a very quick rate especially soon after the surgery is completed, or complications with the gastric band itself which include leaking, loosening, or falling out of place. This can result in infection, and may require further surgery to correct the problem.

With gastric bypass, the body's ability to absorb nutrients is changed drastically, so there is a risk of calcium or iron deficiency which can lead to conditions such as anemia or osteoporosis. Another possible side effect of gastric bypass surgery is dumping syndrome, or the food passing from the stomach to the intestines too quickly without proper digestion, causing pain, nausea, bloating, weakness, or diarrhea. Infections, blood clots, hernia, and gallstones are other side effects of gastric bypass.

With electric devices such as the Maestro system, side effects may include chest pain, nausea, heartburn, vomiting, or belching. There are also certain surgical complication risks and the danger of infection, although the Maestro system is the least invasive of the weight loss surgeries. The device may also have to be reprogrammed by a physician or surgeon if it is inadvertently drained of battery power (the device has to be charged weekly).

Gastric sleeve surgery

Gastric sleeve surgery, also called sleeve gastrectomy, has become popular in recent years as studies have emerged showing its effectivity in weight loss without the complications brought about by gastric bands in other procedures. Gastric sleeve surgery involves removing a large part of your stomach, up to half of its original size, leaving behind a thin vertical sleeve or tube and held together by surgical staples. The procedure is non-reversible.

A sleeve gastrectomy may be performed with the use of a large abdominal incision or open procedure, or by utilizing smaller incisions, a camera, and small surgical instruments (otherwise known as laparoscopic procedure). In many cases, the gastric sleeve surgery is performed by surgeons as the first step of the patient's duodenal switch surgery or gastric bypass, done after about a year. For many patients, the gastric sleeve surgery already delivers significant weight loss and a second procedure is no longer required.

Dr. Kevin McGill, a general and bariatric surgeon at Piedmont Atlanta Hospital, explains, "We leave the patient with a very narrow stomach that's inelastic. What we like about this operation is it's not quite as complex as a gastric bypass."

Also an advantage of gastric sleeve surgery is it removes the part of the stomach that actually produces the hunger hormone known as ghrelin, so the patient will feel less hunger pangs or cravings. "Now, not only can you not eat a lot, but your brain is okay with that," says Dr. McGill. "You don't have those same satiety factors floating around."

Over the last decade, insurance companies have added gastric sleeve surgery to their list of approved or covered weight loss surgeries. Sleeve gastrectomy is now the fastest growing bariatric surgical procedure, with surgeons recommending the operation because of its relatively low complication rates and significant weight loss in patients who have undergone the procedure. The surgery also took less time to complete and was easier to perform, so more surgeons began to recommend it to patients.

At the yearly Obesity Week conference held in November 2015, researchers presented data from more than 70,000 patients who had weight loss surgery between 2010 and 2013. They found that sleeve gastrectomy increased to 49 percent of all weight loss operations performed in 2013, up from only 9 percent in 2010. Meanwhile, gastric bypass procedures decreased from 58 percent of operations in 2010 to 44 percent in 2013.

Why is gastric sleeve surgery less complicated than a gastric bypass? According to Dr. Jaime Ponce, director of bariatric surgery at Dalton Surgical Group in Georgia and former president of American Society for Metabolic and Bariatric Surgery, "The gastric bypass does involve more surgery, because it involves cutting and stapling of the stomach, and rearranging or rerouting the small bowel. So with all that, it's a big surgery that can carry more complications."

On average, a gastric bypass can last around 2 hours, while a sleeve gastrectomy can be performed in an hour or less, so it is more recommended for older patients who may not be ready for a longer medical procedure.

Dr. Linda Zhang, assistant professor of surgery at Mount Sinai Hospital, particularly recommends the gastric sleeve surgery for patients who have tried so many other methods. "Most patients say, 'I've been struggling with weight my whole life — I lose some, then I gain it back. I'm sick of it, and I don't know what to do,' " she says. "With sleeve gastrectomy, I can tell them: This is a surgery where you can lose the weight, maintain the weight loss, and feel more energetic afterward."

The weight loss results for most patients who undergo this procedure are quite remarkable, according to Dr. Zhang. "People can lose up to 70% of their excess body weight — anywhere from 50 to 200 pounds. Postoperatively, patients are on pureed foods for the first three weeks, and then they go back onto regular food. They have to eat extremely small portions and chew very well."

A positive and renewed exuberance may also be brought about by sleeve gastrectomy, especially as patients experience a healthier, more active lifestyle where they have more freedom to enjoy activities they may not have been able to do before the procedure. "A lot of people say that they want the surgery because they want to live longer, and it's shown that this surgery decreases long-term mortality," Dr. Zhang says. "But what shocks people is all the things they can do that they couldn't do before. They tell me they feel more alive and energetic."

Timeline

Your physician or surgeon will assess if a gastric sleeve procedure is the best one for your needs, and if it will be part of a two-step weight loss surgical procedure. Your physician or surgeon will go over the details of the sleeve gastrectomy, the risks associated with the procedure, and what will be required of you prior to the procedure. This would also include diet and physical activity changes you will have to be aware of before and after the surgery.

Once it is assessed that you are ready for sleeve gastrectomy, you will be scheduled for the procedure, depending on the hospital schedule and the availability of the surgeon. Before the operation, you will also need to follow a two-week pre-operation diet, with the primary focus on preparing your body, particularly your liver, for the surgical operation. Keep in mind that if you are obese, your liver is also larger than its normal size, so it has to be reduced in size prior to your gastric sleeve surgery to avoid complications.

Typically, 2-week pre-op diets focus on increasing your protein consumption through eating lean meats, while lowering your carbohydrate consumption by avoiding pasta, rice, breads, cereals, etc. Sugar is also drastically reduced during the two-week pre-op diet, so this means no sugary drinks, juices, candy, chocolate, and desserts.

Many surgeons will also ask you to avoid caffeine two to three days before your gastric sleeve surgery, and to switch to a strict clear liquid diet at least two days before the procedure. A clear liquid diet may consist of broth, water, protein shake, sugar-free Jell-O, sugar-free popsicles, and other similar approved items.

It is very important at this stage to follow your doctor's instructions especially when it comes to what you can and cannot eat, and also when to eat. It is standard for patients about to undergo surgical procedures such as gastric sleeve surgery to avoid consuming any food after midnight of the day before the operation. If you do not adhere to this, your surgery may get cancelled, or there is a greater risk of pulmonary aspiration (vomiting during the operation).

On the day of the surgery, you will go to the pre-operation area where you will be briefed by personnel and meet your anesthesiologist and attending nurse. Paperwork to be filled out, such as consent forms, are completed here. You will also change to your hospital gown and be asked to remove all articles of clothing as well as accessories, such as jewelry, watch, etc.

When all is ready, you will be administered anesthesia. When you wake up after the gastric sleeve surgery, you will already be in the recovery room or your hospital room for the night. It is common for patients to be encouraged to walk a few steps within hours after surgery to avoid blood clots and shoulder pain.

As you are recovering from gastric sleeve surgery, there will now be phases you will have to undergo to ensure full recovery and a successful gastric sleeve surgery. Depending on the operation you underwent, as well as any pain you may be feeling after the surgery, you may stay only one day at the hospital before being discharged, or stay for up to 3 days before getting the clearance from your doctor to go home.

During the recovery time, be sure you are always well-hydrated. Your physician will also let you know what liquids are approved, so make sure to pay attention and always drink enough fluids. You may have to drink slower than normal, or use a drinking straw, but whatever you have to do, just make sure you are drinking your liquids regularly.

Your first week after the operation may also be a difficult time for bowel movements. This is quite normal for most patients after gastric sleeve surgery. Constipation may be experienced during this period as well. If there are other bowel movement issues, make sure to tell your doctor right away so these can be addressed.

If you are taking any prescription medication for other conditions, these drugs may be resumed after the surgery unless otherwise directed by your physician. Time-released medication, if all possible, should be switched to non-time released. All non-time released prescription medication will have to be crushed before ingestion. You will also be prescribed pain medication, and possibly Protonix to control the acidity level in your stomach after the operation.

An important part of the recovery period is your physical activity. Within 5-6 hours after your gastric sleeve surgery, your physician or attending nurse will encourage you to get up and take a few steps, and then increase your walks as the days progress. Walking around prevents blood clots and also speeds up the healing process in your body, while also allowing you to return to normal activities as soon as possible.

Keep in mind that the changes do not end when you are fully healed from the sleeve gastrectomy. Exercise and various forms of physical activity will have to be introduced to your daily lifestyle as part of a healthier transformation, especially if the purpose of the sleeve gastrectomy is to help you lose more weight for another surgical procedure a few months down the road. Getting used to walking during your recovery phase will get you on the mindset of exercise and physical activity.

On the other hand, you would want to avoid excessively strenuous physical activities while you are still in the healing stage, including lifting very heavy things. Your stitches are still new at this point, and your body is still adjusting to the changes so too much physical activity may put undue pressure on your system, causing injury or complications. Because you are consuming less calories, you will feel fatigued for a few weeks after the operation, so it is best to avoid excessive physical exertion.

If you experience any pain that increases in intensity or duration over time, you should immediately contact your physician or hospital so it can be checked right away. You should also seek medical attention right away if you notice red spots, warmth, or pus in the incision area, or if you have a fever, shaking, or chills, especially if your body temperature reaches 101 degrees or higher. If your nausea or vomiting continues for a few days during your healing process, tell your doctor right away.

Diet changes

As you start recovering from gastric sleeve surgery, it is of utmost importance that you understand and adhere to the dietary guidelines which will be given by your physician or dietician. Now that your stomach is smaller, you can only consume a limited amount of food, less than what you have been accustomed to. This means you will have to choose nutrient-dense foods, or foods that are packed with the vitamins and minerals that you need but in controlled amounts, foregoing processed and less-healthy foods that only fill your stomach but do not provide proper nourishment.

The Western lifestyle permeates the idea that bigger is better, and in grocery aisles and restaurants, modern consumers have become lulled to the idea that more food means more health and nourishment. On the contrary, the average supermarket shelf or restaurant menu is full of food offerings that may satisfy hunger pangs but do not provide the balanced nutrition that the person needs. Instead, harmful preservatives, chemicals, and abundance of trans fats, cholesterol, and unnecessary calories are ingested.

With gastric sleeve surgery, the patient is now forced to look closely at meal plans and dietary restrictions because space in the stomach is vastly limited. You will have to carefully assess, with the help of your physician or dietician, which nutrients are needed by your body and in what amounts, and from which food sources to obtain these nutrients from. If you are used to large servings and multiple snack and meal times on a given day, this will all have to change.

It is noteworthy that after sleeve gastrectomy, you will likely not have any desire to eat food because the hunger hormone ghrelin is no longer being produced in your stomach. Because of this change happening in your body, it would be the opportune time to begin getting used to a healthier, more nourishing routine as far as your eating habits go.

During the first week after your operation, you will likely be on a clear liquid diet. The stomach is still healing and cannot handle even soft foods, much less solid foods, so only liquids that are sugar-free may be consumed. This would include water, Jell-O, broth, decaffeinated tea or coffee, sugar-free drinks (check with your doctor first), and sugar-free popsicles. Carbonated and caffeinated drinks are to be avoided.

As you move into the second week post-surgery, full liquids with protein may be introduced aside from the clear liquids you were already consuming the first week. Your doctor may now approve items such as soup with soft noodles, nonfat yogurt, sugar-free pudding or sorbet, sugar-free and zero-fat ice cream, protein powder mix, hot oatmeal or Carnation instant breakfast (sugar-free variant), thinned soups or applesauce, or diluted juices.

On the third week, soft and pureed foods may be introduced to your diet on the advice of your surgeon. Note that food may taste differently than before, even food items you are already used to eating, so take the time to get used to all the changes. During this period, your goal is to reach the recommended protein intake of about 60 grams per day to help you regain your strength. You can start with protein shakes (1 per day, blended with skim milk or yogurt), almond milk or coconut milk (also great for shakes), cottage cheese, hummus, soft cereals and vegetables, ground beef or ground chicken, scrambled egg, steamed fish, canned tuna and salmon, mashed fruits, and other soft or pureed foods with low sugar.

You should still avoid food items that are high in sugar, or starchy and processed foods such as breads, rice, and pasta.

Fibrous vegetables like broccoli, celery, asparagus, and raw leafy greens should also be avoided, as your stomach may not be ready to digest them just yet.

On the fourth week after your surgery, your surgeon will now recommend the introduction of more foods to your diet, but it is important to remember that the stomach is still sensitive and healing at this stage. Therefore, softer versions of food must be prioritized (for instance, mashed or baked potatoes, ground beef or well-cooked chicken) if possible. Also, always remember to chew your food thoroughly. Fish, chicken, and beef may now be eaten, as well as fruits and vegetables that are not fibrous.

During week 4, you should still continue to drink a lot of liquids, especially protein shakes. Caffeine may also be introduced at this stage but very limited. You should still stay away from sodas and high-sugar carbonated drinks, fried foods, candy and chocolate, high carbohydrate food items, and nuts. On the other hand, oatmeal, hard boiled egg, hummus, and fruit cups are recommended especially at breakfast or as healthy snacks.

Beyond the first month, it is highly advisable to stay away from carbonated drinks completely, as these fill up your stomach pretty quickly without providing any nutritional content. Again, remember that your storage space is now limited, so you need to be choosing foods and drinks that pack a lot of punch nutritionally. Even your snacks in between meals should be healthy; for instance, an apple or banana makes for a much better snack item than bread or pasta.

Exercise would be another component at this stage. Start getting into moderate physical activities and exercises such as walking, jogging, swimming, biking and other activities. If you are more into sports and recreational activities, be sure to check with your physician first regarding which sports you should be okay to play again. Those who prefer going to the gym for workouts should also check with their surgeon to make sure it is alright.

Hydration is also very important after you have had your sleeve gastrectomy, so find a reusable water bottle you can carry with you and refill at all times. Throughout the day, keep yourself hydrated and drink regularly even when you are not feeling particularly thirsty. But avoid drinking water during meals, as you want to save the space in your stomach for the food you will consume. Stop drinking water at least a half hour before mealtime so you don't feel full right away.

Carbonated beverages should be a thing of the past after your sleeve gastrectomy. Sodas contain a lot of sugar that you don't need and can set you back in your health goals. Also, the carbonation in sodas can put unnecessary and excessive pressure on your stomach, causing it to stretch. There are plenty of drinks you can substitute for carbonated beverages, such as fruit juices (natural and unsweetened), coconut water, or smoothies (watch out for the sugar content).

Eating three small meals everyday is the best routine for you to pick up after gastric sleeve surgery. Many people skip breakfast, for instance, because they are busy heading to work or other errands in the morning, and then try to make up for it by eating a heavy brunch or lunch. If this is something you are used to doing, be prepared to change this habit. Your meals should be as regular as they are nutritious, and you will have to get used to a regimen of smaller but more nourishing meals.

During check-ups and follow-up sessions with your surgeon or physician, vitamin supplements may be recommended and these supplements should also be adhered to regularly. Your body is adjusting to all of these dietary changes at this point in time, and it needs as much nutrients as possible to stay healthy. Also, you may not be getting as much vitamins, minerals, and other nutrients yet from your new diet plan, so supplements would be an excellent support for your body.

Emotional changes

The reason why physicians and surgeons conduct several counseling sessions and assessments with a patient first before recommending any weight loss surgical procedure such as gastric sleeve surgery is because aside from the physical changes, there are also emotional and psychological changes that the patient will or may undergo. Preparation for different emotional and psychological challenges is just as important before and after the surgical procedure.

Your mental resolve and stability will be put to the test even before the surgery itself, starting with the two-week post-op diet. For many individuals, those changes in dietary consumption would be enough to make them give up already. How committed are you personally to making this positive change in yourself? The many requirements for a successful sleeve gastrectomy will show you just how dedicated you will have to be to this new phase in your life.

The changes don't have to be daunting, however. With the many responsibilities you will have to step up to such as making healthier and more nutritious food choices, being physically active, and avoiding bad habits, you will notice improvements in your weight, energy levels, and overall disposition. Once you see your efforts paying off, this will encourage you to push yourself even further and continue making great strides towards a healthier you.

Even though you have many restrictions as far as diet and lifestyle after your gastric sleeve surgery, it certainly does not mean you will have to give up enjoying your life completely. In fact, the opposite will be more likely, as you will be more energetic and active, and able to enjoy more activities with your family and friends because of a renewed sense of vigor and physical strength. All you will need to do is plan ahead so you can still adhere to your post-surgery dietary restrictions even if you are not at home.

For example, if you have been invited to a friend's house for a dinner party, politely ask what the food choices would be, so you will know if there is something you can enjoy. Most likely, if your friend or family member knows that you have just undergone the procedure and what your diet requirements are, they can make changes to the menu so you can also enjoy the food. If this is not possible, have an alternative plan such as bringing your own food (maybe suggest a potluck instead) or eating your dinner before leaving the house (and just partaking of fruit or other approved items when you get to the party).

When you eat out at a restaurant, be very aware of the ingredients used as well as sugar, fats, calories, and other important information. Most restaurants will allow you to order a half serving of their dishes, so you don't have to worry about eating too much. You will probably get a discount as well if you order only a half portion. This way, you can still enjoy but you are sticking to your nutrition goals at the same time.

One of the most obvious ways you can help yourself is to keep only nutrient-dense snacks and food items in your home. If you are still buying junk food when you go to the grocery store (even if it is for other household members), the urge to partake will be hard to resist because it is readily available. On the other hand, if you only stock nutrient-dense snacks at the house, such as fruit cups, carrot sticks, smoothies, mixed nuts, or fat-free yogurt, you will soon get used to these items as your snack options in between meals.

Speaking of snacks, be careful not to indulge in too much snacks as well, because this can limit your appetite for the more nourishing meals. Your stomach is smaller so even an apple or a cup of yogurt eaten too close to lunch or dinner may make you too full to finish your meal. Try not to get used to snacks in between meal times except if you are really, really hungry. For some people, snacking is just a mental urge, but the body is not really hungry and in need of food in between meals.

Because weight loss will occur after gastric sleeve surgery, hormone production in your body will also be drastically affected. Specifically, levels of estrogen or testosterone may be lower than usual as the body adjusts to the changes. This can result in mood swings or irritability, and other changes in your personality or disposition. Keep in mind that these changes are only temporary and should be manageable. You do want to inform your family or friends, especially those who live with you, about these possible changes.

It is also common for individuals post-surgery to feel tired or fatigued all the time, and this can also cause some mood swings or unpleasantness. The fatigue can cause you to be irritable and to not want to be around people for certain periods of time. Just be patient through the emotional ups and downs after your sleeve gastrectomy. Over time, your mood swings will fade as your body adjusts to the new reality and recovers from the operation, and your disposition should also return to normal.

Lactose intolerance after surgery

One change that you may or may not experience after gastric sleeve surgery is lactose intolerance, or the body's aversion to milk products because of low levels of the enzyme lactase in the small intestine. Lactose intolerance causes the patient to have diarrhea, abdominal pain, or bloating when ingesting milk products with lactose. For patients who were not lactose intolerant prior to the operation, this can be a surprising reality to handle. The great thing is there are ways to deal with lactose intolerance after gastric sleeve surgery.

If you find that you are lactose intolerant after the procedure, inform your doctor or dietician right away so they can guide you on what steps to take regarding this. Usually, you will be advised to consume milk products very slowly at a time and in very minimal amounts first to give the body time to adjust.

According to Pam Davis, a certified bariatric nurse at the TriStar Centennial Center for Weight Management in Nashville, Tennessee, if the patient was already lactose intolerant before the procedure, then those issues would pop up. She adds, "Individuals without previous history of lactose intolerance ... may find themselves experiencing a transient period of lactose intolerance that begins once the patient is on the full liquid stage of the diet. There will be a percentage of patients who continue to experience lactose intolerance long-term. For those individuals, we've found the fast-acting Lactaid tablets taken with the first bite of food can help minimize symptoms."

Meanwhile, Linda Steakley, a dietitian from the Huntsville Wellness Center in Alabama, recommends cheese and Greek yogurt as alternative sources of protein, calcium and Vitamin D for patients with lactose intolerance after gastric sleeve surgery. "Cheese is naturally low in lactose as a protein dairy source if a patient has an inability to digest milk properly after surgery. Another good source of protein comes from yogurt."

Steakley adds, "Greek yogurt is especially high in protein. Not only are we concerned about their protein intakes but calcium and vitamin D are critical to the bariatric patient in order to reduce their chances of developing osteoporosis."

Goodbye artificial/processed foods

As already mentioned, now that you have a smaller stomach you need to make wise choices as far as what food to consume, considering you have a more limited space and must make the most of it. With this in mind, your goal should always be to eliminate processed or artificial foods from your meals and snacks, and focus instead on nourishing your body with nutrient-dense whole foods that deliver the most vitamins and minerals but with less calories.

Choosing nutrient-dense whole foods over processed foods makes a lot more sense when you make a comparison between the two. Let's take, for instance, the case between white bread and whole wheat bread. One slice of white bread and whole wheat bread both have essentially the same number of calories (around 80 calories). But one slice of white bread only contains less than 1 mg of vitamin E, while a slice of whole wheat bread contains up to 500 mg of the same vitamin.

The average Western diet is chock full of processed food items such as pasta, microwave dinners, French fries, burgers, potato chips, soda, candy, chocolate, breads, pastries, and other foods that can hinder you from reaching optimal health after your gastric sleeve surgery. If you want to make the most of the operation, and also avoid problems with recovery or weight maintenance after your procedure, you should switch to healthy food fare such as fruits and vegetables, whole grains, fat-free or low-fat dairy, seafood, lean poultry, lean meats, eggs, beans, nuts, and very limited amounts of fats, sugars, trans fats, cholesterol, salt, and saturated fats.

Of course, it is a must to always communicate and work with your doctor or dietitian when it comes to the foods you will eat after sleeve gastrectomy. They will be the best people to determine what you should and should not eat, depending on your recovery and progress. For example, while vegetables are generally good for you as you transform your diet, fibrous vegetables must be avoided within the first four weeks after your gastric sleeve procedure.

Positive changes will be apparent within the first few weeks after your operation and as you adopt healthier food choices, but it is inevitable to also waver in your resolve at times and want to revert back to your old ways. Just remember to keep your perspective in the long-term; it may not be as fun or sexy right now to stick to the diet or meal plans prepared for you by your doctor and/or your dietitian, but in the long run these changes will help you in your health and fitness goals.

Have a support group

A support group providing assistance and accountability may be beneficial for you as well. There are plenty of support networks, peer groups, and volunteer associations that your doctor or dietitian may be able to refer you to. These groups are ideally made up of people who are also going through or have gone through the same challenges and experiences as yours, and can provide much-needed encouragement and advice as you take on this journey.

Accountability is also important especially as you recover from the gastric sleeve surgery, with various dietary changes that need to be fulfilled as you recover from the procedure. If you are finding it difficult to relate with family members or friends regarding your condition as well as your need for accountability and affirmation, reach out to a support group in your area that can fill the void for you.

The importance of recipes

When starting a new regimen or routine, whether it is a diet or meal plan, an exercise or workout plan, or a new outdoor activity or sport, you will need some time to learn the ropes and settle into a rhythm that is comfortable and manageable for your system. The learning does not stop, of course, as there will always be new information to take in and new facets of the activity to learn. But once you have set the foundation, following through with this new regimen will be more attainable especially as you become more accustomed to all the tasks entailed.

As you seek to change your eating habits and become a stronger, healthier version of yourself after your gastric sleeve surgery, you would benefit greatly from a structured, well-planned set of meal plans and easy-to-follow recipes that address the nutritional needs that have to be met, while also allowing you to enjoy different variety and some room for mixing and matching. If you already have recipes on hand, this will lessen your time and effort in looking at different sources for appropriate meal ideas in line with your health and fitness goals.

Recipes provide you with guidance on what to purchase when you are at the grocery store. Because you are following a meal plan, you will be constantly reminded to look for the ingredients that you will need to prepare the suggested recipes. On the other hand, without the guidance of a written or printed recipe, you will likely waste a lot of time and effort figuring out what to buy, and end up buying food items you actually do not need. Recipes keep your food shopping in check.

Another advantage of having meal plans and recipes is the information it can readily provide to your doctor or dietitian regarding your nutritional intake and what may need to be changed. For example, if you come in for a checkup one day and the physician notices that you are lacking vitamin D, he can take a look at the recipes or meal plans that you are following, and then immediately take note of where changes can be made. This is more time efficient than having to ask you to remember what you have been eating the last two weeks.

If you are a homemaker, then you probably already know how stressful it can be to think of meals to prepare everyday for the household. Family members want variety, and you have to come up with meal ideas that your loved ones are not tired of just yet. Otherwise, it will come down to preparing home cooked meals on certain days of the week, and then eating out or buying food for the other days.

As you recover from gastric sleeve surgery, you would want at least this step of thinking and preparing for meals to be the least of your concerns. After all, you have other things in your mind and you should not end up stressing yourself out with details that can very well be ironed out ahead of time. Recipes and meal plans are helpful in this regard. They lessen the time you need to devote to figuring out what to eat. Instead, all you will need to do is refer to the guide for assistance.

Recipes also save you money. The ingredients you will need (and the amounts) are already listed down for you, and this gives you an idea how much to buy. This eliminates unnecessary spending on food items that you should not even purchase in the first place. Also, a meal plan or recipe for each day of the week will minimize the instances when you have to order in or get take out food. Obviously, meals prepared at home are cheaper than those bought outside, so you also get savings.

Following recipes and meal plans makes it easier for you to make healthier food fare choices. If you know what fruits, vegetables, meat products, and other items you will need for the week, you can plan on purchasing the ingredients at a local organic store, for instance. Remember that your goal is to consume nutrient-dense foods after your sleeve gastrectomy, and organic and whole foods are definitely better choices than most commercially- or mass-produced foods.

In the next few chapters, you will find recipes that are easy to prepare, cost-efficient, and provide variety to your meal times. Granted, these recipes may not necessarily be what you have been used to eating for most of your life. But these recipes and meal plans can greatly assist you with getting back to your optimum self after gastric sleeve surgery, and providing you with the right nutrients you need as you reach your fitness goals.

The recipes provided in the following chapters of this eBook are not complicated. They are very easy to follow, whether you are an experienced cook or just starting out. If you have never had the time or the patience to prepare meals at home, now may be the best time to start. Preparing your own meals gives you the assurance that the ingredients you are using contain the most nutrients that your body requires.

The beauty of recipes is they are easy to tweak or revise according to your needs or specifications. If you find some areas for improvement or just want to change things up a bit, you are more than welcome to do so because it is your meal preparation after all. As you are preparing your meals, you are also getting in the mindset of changing more and more aspects of your personal life towards self-improvement and better health.

The recipes that will be presented in this eBook are mainly for the fluid and soft food stage after your gastric sleeve surgery. Details regarding preparation time, cooking time, ingredients, serving information, nutritional content, and alteration options will be presented, so you will have all the necessary knowledge to follow the plans.

More recipes for the solid food stage will be presented under the same series. You can stay updated by signing up for our newsletter.

Part II Understanding the Fluid Stage and Soft Food Stage

Stage 1: Fluid (including Clear Fluid and Full Fluid with Protein)

Sleeve gastrectomy is designed to help you lose weight by reducing the size of your stomach, thereby reducing the amount of food you can consume. Also, another effect of sleeve gastrectomy is limiting the production of the hunger hormone called ghrelin. When this hormone is no longer present or being produced in your stomach, the hunger pangs or cravings are drastically reduced.

It is important to note, however, that gastric sleeve surgery, or any other weight loss surgery, does not automatically guarantee that you will lose weight. It is just the first step towards your goal of becoming healthy and fit. Gastric sleeve surgery is just one procedure that can make the goal of optimum health more attainable for patients, but it is not the end-all and be-all solution. It is a major boost to the effort, but you will also have to put in your part.

As already mentioned in the previous chapter, changes in your diet and lifestyle have to be strictly adhered to if you want to see any significant positive results from your gastric sleeve surgery. It is not just the weight loss results, however, that you should keep in mind when following the recommended dietary restrictions after your sleeve gastrectomy. During your first two weeks post-operation, the stomach is still recovering. Deviating from the prescribed dietary guidelines could result in complications and other problems.

If you do not follow your doctor's orders to the last syllable, some complications that could arise include dehydration, diarrhea, constipation, bowel obstruction, or a gastric leak which could be very troublesome as you have just finished the surgery. So listen and understand the information which your doctor and/or surgeon will give you, and don't attempt to cheat.

Stage 1a: Clear liquids

On the week immediately preceding the sleeve gastrectomy, you will be restricted to a diet consisting of clear liquids only. This may sound like a very difficult undertaking, but remember that during the surgical procedure, the part of your stomach which produces ghrelin is removed, so the usual hunger pangs you feel will not be there during the first week. This will make the clear liquid diet a little easier to maintain.

On the clear liquid diet, the following items are approved: water, broth, Jell-O (sugar-free), decaffeinated tea, decaffeinated coffee, non-carbonated sugar-free drinks, and sugar-free popsicles. Your doctor or dietitian may have other suggestions in mind, so be sure to check with them. Meanwhile, to be avoided during the first week after the surgical operation would be the following: caffeinated drinks, carbonated drinks, sugary drinks.

During this stage, take small sips of the fluids you are taking. Try to avoid using drinking straws or drinking bottles as these can cause gas bubbles. Be aware of any signs of fullness during this period. Also, most fruit juices are okay to drink as long they are unsweetened (apple juice or orange juice) but make sure you are getting the fresh or unprocessed brands. If you can get them freshly-squeezed or extracted, much better.

The clear liquid stage will be a determining factor of your recovery. If your body is able to tolerate water and other clear liquids during the first week, then you will be able to move on to full fluids with protein the following week. Mostly, the clear fluids are administered to keep you hydrated while the body, especially the stomach area, is healing and getting stronger after the gastric sleeve surgery.

Stage 1b: Full fluid with protein

On the second week after your sleeve gastrectomy, full fluids with protein may be introduced slowly. Full liquids should be smooth in texture and with liquid consistency, without any seeds or lumps. It is also advised during this stage of the recovery process to take small sips at a time, taking note of any feelings of fullness and avoiding undue pressure on the stomach. Clear liquids from the first week may still be taken at this time.

At this stage, the goal is to nourish your body with much-needed protein from approved sources. The protein is needed to improve your strength and speed up the healing and recovery process. Approved foods would include: protein powder mix, pudding (sugar-free), soups, non-fat yogurt, hot oatmeal (low or no sugar), thinned applesauce, protein shakes (with approximately 20 grams of protein per serving, less than 10 grams of sugar per serving, less than 200 calories per serving), low fat or light soy milk, and other full fluids.

For the long-term, even after you have fully healed and are able to consume solid foods again, protein shakes in particular should be considered as a staple in your health and fitness goals. Protein shakes provide much-needed nourishment without too much calories, and there are many varieties you can choose from. Protein shakes are also quite easy to prepare, and can keep you feeling full especially when there are cravings.

Dehydration should still be prevented at this stage. Your doctor or dietitian may recommend up to eight cups of caffeine-free and low-calorie liquids taken throughout the day in between meals. It would normally be recommended not to drink during meals as well, and to wait up to 45 minutes after meals before drinking fluids again.

If you do not have a blender, it is best to purchase one before your gastric sleeve surgery. There are many approved foods with much-needed protein and other essential nutrients that you can blenderize for consumption on the weeks following the procedure, all towards the goal of at least 72 grams of protein per day.

Non-fat or skim milk is another dairy product you would want to make a regular in your diet. It contains the protein you need for your body but without the unnecessary fat. A cup of skim milk (or about 8 ounces) is packed with calcium and vitamin D (up to 30% of your daily needed intake), but also other important nutrients such as protein, riboflavin, niacin, and phosphorus. Aside from drinking skim milk, you can also consume it with your cereal

Almond milk and coconut milk are becoming popular among the health conscious as well, and if you have not tried these yet, you can add them to your diet. Almond milk, in particular, is low in fat and has lots of proteins, fiber, and lipids, as well as potassium, sodium, zinc, calcium, iron magnesium, vitamins C and B6, thiamine, niacin, riboflavin, folate, and vitamin E. Almond milk improves your heart health and keeps your bones strong, both components which you will need to keep healthy as you try to adopt a more active lifestyle after your gastric sleeve surgery. You can purchase almond milk from most stores (ask your dietitian for recommended brands), or you can even prepare almond milk at home (yet another reason to purchase a blender).

Coconut milk, meanwhile, is a great substitute for cow's milk if you experience lactose intolerance after sleeve gastrectomy. Coconut milk does not contain lactose, and is also popular among vegetarians and vegans. It can be used for cooking, baking, or with your protein shakes and fruit smoothies. One 100ml serving of coconut milk will give you 1.4 grams of protein, 15 grams of fat, 3.4 grams of carbohydrates, and other essential nutrients such as fiber, vitamins C and E, all the B vitamins, magnesium, selenium, and phosphorus.

Stage 2: Soft Food

As your body is recovering from the sleeve gastrectomy, your doctor or dietitian may recommend that you start introducing soft, pureed foods to your diet on the third week after the operation. You can still continue consuming clear liquids and full fluids with protein from the previous weeks, but now you can also add more food items to your diet while also adding nourishment to your body.

On the third week, it is important to remember that your protein intake goal is at least 60 grams per day (if you can get up to 70 grams per day that would be more beneficial). Also, don't rush your meals. Sip your pureed foods slowly to give you stomach time to adjust. Remember that at this point your stomach has not digested anything more than clear and full liquids so it will take some getting used to the new foods in your diet all over again.

You may notice that some foods you were used to eating in the past, even staples such as meats, dairy, vegetables, or fruits, taste differently than they did. This is because there are a lot of changes going in your body, so give it some time and be patient in slowly introducing foods to your system. Take note of foods or drinks that cause stomach upsets, diarrhea, or gas so you can avoid or limit them for the time being.

Approved foods at this stage include: soups with blenderized meats (no lumps), scrambled eggs, cottage cheese, cereal, boiled chicken, fish, mashed potatoes, protein shakes, and lots of other blenderized or pureed foods you can tolerate. On the other hand, stay away from smoothies that have way too much sugar, starchy items such as bread or pasta, and fibrous vegetables including broccoli and asparagus.

Because your goal is weight loss, opt for low-fat varieties as much as possible, such as low-fat cottage cheese. Other cheeses are alright to consume in moderate amounts, but don't overeat them because cheeses are usually high in fat. 100 grams of cottage cheese typically contains 3 grams of carbohydrates, 11 grams of protein, and plenty of vitamins A and D, selenium, zinc, calcium, potassium, iron, sodium, magnesium, and phosphorus, while only containing 4.5 grams of fat.

Vegetables may be steamed or boiled at this stage to make them softer and easier to eat. The typical Western diet does not include enough vegetables, so this is something you will have to incorporate in your diet. Once you get used to eating vegetables every day and you see the positive effects, you will see how important they are to maintaining good health and helping you with your weight loss goals.

The majority of vegetables have low calories and fat, so you can consume what you need without worrying about your weight. Also, vegetables do not contain cholesterol, so if you are eating them without sauces or seasonings, you are not consuming any cholesterol at all. As your body is healing after sleeve gastrectomy, it will need the vitamin C provided by vegetables, vitamin A to protect against infections, and potassium for normal blood pressure.

Another excellent addition to your soft food diet is canned fish, including tuna and salmon. Canned tuna is relatively inexpensive and easy to purchase, but make sure to ask your dietitian or doctor for recommended brands. Canned tuna provides lean protein which your body needs at this point; a single 4-ounce serving of canned tuna contains 30 grams of protein and all 10 essential amino acids. A word of caution: canned tuna contains high amounts of sodium or salt, so limit your other sodium intake and only consume canned tuna in moderation.

Canned salmon is rich in calcium, iron, unsaturated or healthy fats, and protein (a ¼ cup serving of canned salmon contains 12 grams of protein). You can eat canned salmon straight out of the can, or add it other meals and dishes. Depending on where you live, you may actually find that fresh salmon (along with tuna and other types of fish) is actually easier to buy and cheaper than the canned varieties, so check out your local markets and organic stores first. Also, ask a health professional for recommended brands with lower sodium content.

Most people already know that fruits are excellent for the health, but not everyone still gets enough fruit servings in their diet. Fruits contain little fat, sodium, and calories, so they are great for your fitness goals after gastric sleeve surgery. You do need to watch out for the sugar content in many fruits, but as long as you do not overeat this should not be much of a problem. What you do want is the generous amounts of antioxidants and other nutrients that fruits contain.

In particular, some of the very important nutrients that a lot of people are not getting as much but can get from fruits include vitamin C, folate, potassium, and dietary fiber. Fruits help to keep your heart healthy, and also aid in fast healing and recovery, so you will need your fruit intake to boost your body's healing stage after sleeve gastrectomy. The dietary fiber in fruits will also keep your bowel movements normal, and aid in weight loss.

Some fruits are great for smoothies and milkshakes (mango, banana, cantaloupe, coconut, apple, papaya, strawberry) so you can prepare them and drink them on the go, in between meals, or even as complete meals themselves. While there are fruits you can also include in cooked or baked food items, it is recommended that you eat many fruits raw or unprocessed in order to get the most phytochemicals, antioxidants, flavonoids, and other nutrients from them.

Specifically recommended for weight loss is the lychee, which acts as a laxative so it helps with your digestive processes but contains few calories and no cholesterol or saturated fats. Other fruits that are great for your weight loss goals include papaya, zucchini, banana, and tomato. Simply adding fruits to your daily diet even after this stage of your post-operation recovery will help you shed those unwanted pounds.

Aside from the food that will be recommended to you by your doctor or dietitian, they may also recommend vitamin or mineral supplements. This may be especially useful in the first month or so after your gastric sleeve surgery. Because you are still adjusting to the smaller stomach size, and the body is also in an adjustment period, there may be deficiencies in some vitamins and minerals needed by your system. However, you may not be getting all of these from foods yet, so supplements may be necessary.

Supplements may also be recommended even after you have fully recovered. No matter what vitamin or mineral supplements you may be taking, it is still important to stick to the recommended diet from your physician or dietitian. Many fruits and vegetables also assist in better absorption of vitamins and minerals from food, so you should still eat them regularly.

FLUID AND PUREE

HIBISCUS ICED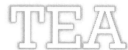

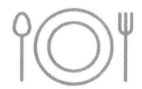

PREP TIME	COOK TIME	SERVES
5 MINUTES	8 HOURS	8

INGREDENTS

1/2 cup dried hibiscus flowers

1 cinnamon stick

4 cups cold water

1 lime, juice only

Stevia to taste

DIRECTIONS

1. In a large Jar, add hibiscus flowers, cinnamon stick and water. Refrigerate overnight.

2. Strain out the solid. Add Lime juice and stevia to taste.

NUTRITION FACTS (PER SERVING)

CALORIES	21	KCal
PROTEIN	<1	g
FAT	<1	g
CARBOHYDRATES	5.6	g
SODIUM	10	mg

FLUID AND PUREE

LIME POPSICLE

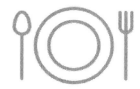

PREP TIME	COOK TIME	SERVES
10 MINUTES	4 HOURS	4

INGREDENTS

3 lime, juice only

1 1/2 cups water

4 packets stevia

DIRECTIONS

1. Add all ingredients in a medium sized bowl. Stir until all powders are dissolved.

2. Pour the mixture into 4 4-oz popsicle molds, dividing equally.

3. Insert sticks and freeze until hardened. About 4 hours.

NUTRITION FACTS (PER SERVING)

CALORIES	11	KCal
PROTEIN	<1	g
FAT	<1	g
CARBOHYDRATES	3.6	g
SODIUM	4	mg

FLUID AND PUREE
CLEAR CHICKEN BROTH

PREP TIME
30 MINUTES

COOK TIME
2 HOURS 15
MINUTES

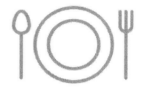

SERVES
26

INGREDENTS

5 chicken legs, skin removed

2 medium onions, peeled and cut into quarters

2 stalks celery, cut into 1-inch pieces

1 large carrot, peeled and cut into 1-inch pieces

2 cloves garlic

5 sprigs fresh parsley

1 teaspoon dried thyme

2 bay leaves

1 1/2 teaspoons salt

DIRECTIONS

1. Place the chicken legs in a soup pot and cover in cold water. Bring it to a boil over high heat.

2. Drain and remove the water. Add water to cover the chicken and use low heat to bring it to a simmer. continue to remove any impurities that rises to the surface until the water is cleared.

3. Add all remaining ingredients. Simmer for 1 hour.

4. Remove the legs. Pull off the meat from the bones with a pair of forks. Add the bones and meats back to the broth. Simmer for another 1 hour.

5. Remove all solid from the broth. Pour the broth through a sieve lined with cheesecloth to remove fine chunks and oil.

6. Set aside to cool and then remove the oil on the surface.

7. Refrigerate for use within 3 days or freeze up to 3 months

Selena's Special Tips:
- *For easy storage, freeze the broth in 4-oz popsicle molds and pop out and store in freezer bags. 1 stick is 1 serving. When needed, microwave 30 seconds before eating.*

NUTRITION FACTS (PER SERVING)

CALORIES	11	KCal
PROTEIN	< 1	g
FAT	< 1	g
CARBOHYDRATES	< 1	g
SODIUM	140	mg

FLUID AND PUREE

CHOCOLATE MOUSSE

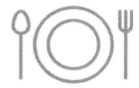

PREP TIME	COOK TIME	SERVES
5 MINUTES	2 HOURS 15 MINUTES	8

INGREDENTS

12 Oz fat-free Greek yogurt

1 / 2 cup unsweetened cocoa powder

3 / 4 cup unsweetened almond milk

1 / 2 cup erythritol

1 / 2 teaspoon vanilla extract

1 / 2 scoop chocolate/vanilla-flavored protein

DIRECTIONS

1. Place cocoa powder, almond milk and erythritol in a saucepan. Heat over medium heat and keep stirring until thickened, about 5 minutes. Set aside to cool.

2. Once cooled, add protein powder (optional) and stir until well incorporated.

3. Add vanilla extract to Greek yogurt. Whisk until fluffy. Add the yogurt to the chocolate mixture and stir until well incorporated.

4. Cover and refrigerate for at least 2.5 hours before serving.

NUTRITION FACTS (PER SERVING)

CALORIES	39	KCal
PROTEIN	4.0	g
FAT	<1	g
CARBOHYDRATES	5.4	g
SODIUM	31	mg

FLUID AND PUREE

LEMON YOGURT POPSICLES

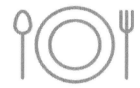

PREP TIME	COOK TIME	SERVES
5 MINUTES	6 HOURS	6

INGREDENTS

22 Oz fat-free Greek yogurt

1 / 4 cup lemon juice

2 tablespoons unsweetened almond milk

3 tablespoons erythritol

DIRECTIONS

1. Combine all ingredients in a large bowl. Taste the mixture. Add extra lemon juice or sweetener if desired.

2. Pour the mixture into 6 4-oz popsicle molds, dividing equally.

3. Insert sticks and freeze until hardened. About 6 hours.

NUTRITION FACTS (PER SERVING)

CALORIES	64	KCal
PROTEIN	11.1	g
FAT	<1	g
CARBOHYDRATES	5.3	g
SODIUM	43	mg

FLUID AND PUREE

VANILLA PEANUT BUTTER 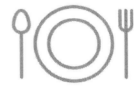 ICE CREAM

PREP TIME
5 MINUTES

COOK TIME
4 HOURS

SERVES
4

INGREDENTS

2 cups unsweetened almond milk

2 scoops vanilla-flavored protein powder

2 tablespoons powdered peanut butter

1/8 teaspoon salt

DIRECTIONS

1. Combine all ingredients in a plastic container

2. Place in the freezer. Whisk the mixture thoroughly every 30 minutes until the ice cream is firm.

NUTRITION FACTS (PER SERVING)

CALORIES	54	KCal
PROTEIN	5.2	g
FAT	2.4	g
CARBOHYDRATES	3.2	g
SODIUM	254	mg

FLUID AND PUREE

CREAM OF BROCCOLI SOUP

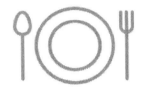

PREP TIME
10 MINUTES

COOK TIME
30 MINUTES

SERVES
12

INGREDENTS

10 Oz low-fat chicken broth

1 1/4 cups water

2 1/4 cups broccoli, chopped including the stems

1/2 cup onion, diced

1/2 cup evaporated skim milk

1/2 cup fat free cheddar cheese, shredded

DIRECTIONS

1. Place broth, water, broccoli and onion in a saucepan and bring it to boil over medium-high heat

2. Reduce to low heat and simmer for 20 minutes

3. Add evaporated skim milk slowly while stirring

4. Add cheese and stir until well-incorporated

5. Remove from the flame and keep aside to cool. Once cooled, blend in a mixer till smooth. Pour it through a mesh lined with a clean cheesecloth to remove chunks

6. Reheat the soup to desired temperature.

7. Dissolve protein powder in 2 tablespoons of water

8. Slowly add the protein mixture while stirring

Selena's Special Tips:

- *Protein power tends to form clumps in hot liquids. Make sure to let the soup cool a bit before adding the mixture.*

NUTRITION FACTS (PER SERVING)

CALORIES	35	KCal
PROTEIN	3.0	g
FAT	1.3	g
CARBOHYDRATES	3.3	g
SODIUM	83	mg

FLUID AND PUREE
PUMPKIN SOUP

PREP TIME
15 MINUTES

COOK TIME
20 minutes

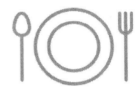

SERVES
18

INGREDENTS

3 cups red pumpkin, cut into 1-inch pieces

1 teaspoon low-fat butter

1/4 cup onion, finely chopped

1 teaspoon dried oregano

1 cup fat-free milk

salt to taste

DIRECTIONS

1. Add butter in a saucepan. Sauté onion for 1 minute over medium heat

2. Add Pumpkin. Sauté for 3 minute

3. Add 3 cups of water. Cover the pan and cook for 10 minutes while stirring occasionally. Add oregano.

4. Set aside to cool. Then blend until smooth. Pour it through a mesh lined with a clean cheesecloth to remove chunks

5. Reheat the mixture and slowly add milk and cook for 3 minutes while stirring. Set aside to cool.

6. Dissolve protein powder in 2 tablespoons of water

7. Slowly add the protein mixture while stirring

Selena's Special Tips:

- *Protein power tends to form clumps in hot liquids. Make sure to let the soup cool a bit before adding the mixture.*

NUTRITION FACTS (PER SERVING)

CALORIES	12	KCal
PROTEIN	<1	g
FAT	<1	g
CARBOHYDRATES	2.2	g
SODIUM	71	mg

FLUID AND PUREE

CHOCOLATE BERRY SMOOTHIE

PREP TIME
5 MINUTES

COOK TIME
5 minutes

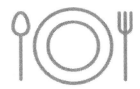

SERVES
1

INGREDENTS

3 **Oz** fat-free Greek yogurt

4 **Oz** ice cubes

1 **scoop** chocolate-flavored protein powder

2 **tablespoons** frozen berry

liquid stevia to taste

DIRECTIONS

1. Blend all ingredients until smooth. Thin with water if
   necessary.

NUTRITION FACTS (PER SERVING)

CALORIES	140	KCal
PROTEIN	19.8	g
FAT	2.1	g
CARBOHYDRATES	7.6	g
SODIUM	188	mg

FLUID AND PUREE
STRAWBERRY DELIGHT

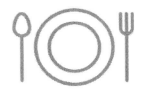

PREP TIME	COOK TIME	SERVES
5 MINUTES	5 minutes	1

INGREDENTS

4 Oz fat-free Greek yogurt

4 Oz ice cubes

1 scoop vanilla-flavored protein powder

1/4 cup frozen strawberry

1/8 teaspoon nutmeg

liquid stevia to taste

DIRECTIONS

1. Blend all ingredients until smooth. Thin with water if necessary.

NUTRITION FACTS (PER SERVING)

CALORIES	128	KCal
PROTEIN	19.5	g
FAT	1.0	g
CARBOHYDRATES	10.2	g
SODIUM	103	mg

FLUID AND PUREE

PUMPKIN PIE SMOOTHIE

PREP TIME
5 MINUTES

COOK TIME
5 minutes

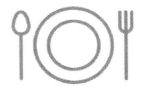

SERVES
1

INGREDENTS

4 Oz fat-free Greek yogurt

4 Oz ice cubes

1 scoop vanilla-flavored protein powder

1/4 cup canned pumpkin

1/4 teaspoon cinnamon

Pinch of pumpkin spices

liquid stevia to taste

DIRECTIONS

1. Blend all ingredients until smooth. Thin with water if necessary.

NUTRITION FACTS (PER SERVING)

CALORIES	136	KCal
PROTEIN	20.2	g
FAT	1.2	g
CARBOHYDRATES	12.0	g
SODIUM	106	mg

FLUID AND PUREE
CHOCOLATE PEANUT BUTTER SHAKE

PREP TIME

5 MINUTES

COOK TIME

5 minutes

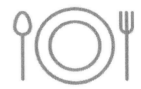

SERVES

1

INGREDENTS

3 Oz fat-free Greek yogurt

4 Oz ice cubes

1 scoop chocolate-flavored protein powder

1 tablespoons powdered peanut butter

liquid stevia to taste

DIRECTIONS

1. Blend all ingredients until smooth. Thin with water if necessary.

NUTRITION FACTS (PER SERVING)

CALORIES	152	KCal
PROTEIN	25.6	g
FAT	2.8	g
CARBOHYDRATES	8.2	g
SODIUM	136	mg

FLUID AND PUREE

APPLE PIE SMOOTHIE

PREP TIME
5 MINUTES

COOK TIME
5 minutes

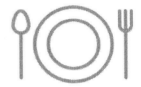

SERVES
1

INGREDENTS

3 1/2 Oz fat-free Greek yogurt

4 Oz ice cubes

1 scoop vanilla-flavored protein powder

1/4 small apple, cubed

1/4 teaspoon cinnamon

Pinch of nutmeg

liquid stevia to taste

70

DIRECTIONS

1. Blend all ingredients until smooth. Thin with water if necessary.

NUTRITION FACTS (PER SERVING)

CALORIES	122	KCal
PROTEIN	18.6	g
FAT	1.1	g
CARBOHYDRATES	10.1	g
SODIUM	100	mg

FLUID AND PUREE

CARROT CAKE SMOOTHIE

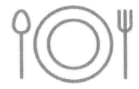

PREP TIME

5 MINUTES

COOK TIME

5 minutes

SERVES

1

INGREDENTS

4 Oz fat-free Greek yogurt

4 Oz ice cubes

1 scoop vanilla-flavored protein powder

1/4 cup canned carrot

1/4 teaspoon vanilla extract

Pinch of cinnamon, ginger, nutmeg

liquid stevia to taste

DIRECTIONS

1. Blend all ingredients until smooth. Thin with water if necessary.

NUTRITION FACTS (PER SERVING)

CALORIES	128	KCal
PROTEIN	19.5	g
FAT	1.0	g
CARBOHYDRATES	10.1	g
SODIUM	123	mg

FLUID AND PUREE

COCONUT DREAM SHAKE

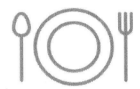

PREP TIME	COOK TIME	SERVES
5 MINUTES	5 minutes	1

INGREDENTS

4 Oz fat-free Greek yogurt

4 Oz ice cubes

1 scoop vanilla-flavored protein powder

1/2 teaspoon coconut extract

1/2 teaspoon vanilla extract

Pinch of nutmeg

liquid stevia to taste

DIRECTIONS

1. Blend all ingredients until smooth. Thin with water if necessary.

NUTRITION FACTS (PER SERVING)

CALORIES	118	KCal
PROTEIN	19.5	g
FAT	1.0	g
CARBOHYDRATES	7.1	g
SODIUM	103	mg

FLUID AND PUREE
RICOTTA PROTEIN PANCAKES

PREP TIME
5 MINUTES

COOK TIME
15 minutes

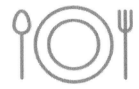

SERVES
1

INGREDENTS

2 **tablespoons** low fat Ricotta cheese

1 **scoop** vanilla-flavored protein powder

1 large egg, white only

1/4 **teaspoon** vanilla extract

1/8 **teaspoon** baking powder

DIRECTIONS

1. Combine all ingredient and whisk thoroughly

2. Pour a small pancake. Cook over medium-low heat until the bottom is slightly firm.

3. Flip and cook for another 20-30 seconds.

NUTRITION FACTS (PER SERVING)

CALORIES	125	KCal
PROTEIN	17.1	g
FAT	3.6	g
CARBOHYDRATES	6.8	g
SODIUM	303	mg

FLUID AND PUREE

ITALIAN TUNA SALAD

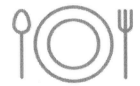

PREP TIME	COOK TIME	SERVES
5 MINUTES	5 minutes	4

INGREDENTS

10 Oz tuna, packed in water, drained

1/4 cup fat free Italian dressing

1 tablespoon lemon juice

DIRECTIONS

1. Mix all ingredients in a large bowl and serve.

NUTRITION FACTS (PER SERVING)

CALORIES	70	KCal
PROTEIN	13.9	g
FAT	0.8	g
CARBOHYDRATES	11.6	g
SODIUM	388	mg

FLUID AND PUREE

LEMON PEPPER COD

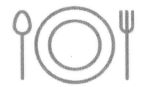

PREP TIME	COOK TIME	SERVES
5 MINUTES	5 minutes	4

INGREDENTS

5 Oz fresh cod fish

1 tablespoon lemon juice

1 teaspoon Mrs. Dash Lemon Pepper Seasoning

Pinch of salt

DIRECTIONS

1. Wash the cod fish with water and lemon juice

2. Season with lemon pepper seasoning and salt

3. Put the fish in a non-stick pan and add a little bit of water

4. Simmer over low heat until cooked.

5. Break down the chunk with a pair of forks before serve

NUTRITION FACTS (PER SERVING)

CALORIES	75	KCal
PROTEIN	16.2	g
FAT	0.6	g
CARBOHYDRATES	0	g
SODIUM	56	mg

FLUID AND PUREE

SALMON YOGURT MOUSSE

PREP TIME
30 MINUTES

COOK TIME
3 HOURS

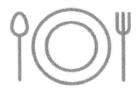

SERVES
4

INGREDENTS

9 Oz salmon, bone and skin removed

4 Oz fat free Greek yogurt

1/4 cup cold water

1 teaspoon gelatin

1 teaspoon fat-free mayonnaise

1 teaspoon onion, grated

1 teaspoon lemon juice

1 / 4 teaspoon dill

pinch of salt

DIRECTIONS

1. Soak the gelatin in the cold water and let it set for 5 minutes

2. Heat the water until the gelatin melts

3. Blend the salmon, yogurt and mayonnaise

4. Add gelatin and the remaining ingredients and mix until well incorporated.

5. Refrigerate for at least 3 hours before serve.

NUTRITION FACTS (PER SERVING)

CALORIES	155	KCal
PROTEIN	25.0	g
FAT	4.9	g
CARBOHYDRATES	1.1	g
SODIUM	101	mg

FLUID AND PUREE

SIMPLE CHICKEN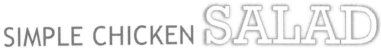

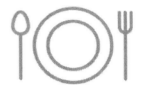

PREP TIME
5 MINUTES

COOK TIME
5 MINUTES

SERVES
1

INGREDENTS

2 Oz chicken breast, cooked and shredded or canned chicken

1 Oz fat free Greek yogurt

1 tablespoon light mayonnaise

salt and pepper to taste

DIRECTIONS

1. Mix all ingredients in a large bowl and serve.

NUTRITION FACTS (PER SERVING)

CALORIES	124	KCal
PROTEIN	20.4	g
FAT	5.5	g
CARBOHYDRATES	11.9	g
SODIUM	172	mg

FLUID AND PUREE

CHICKEN LIME SOUP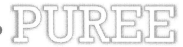

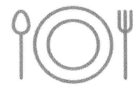

PREP TIME	COOK TIME	SERVES
15 MINUTES	2 HOURS	12

INGREDENTS

1 **pound** boneless skinless chicken breasts

1 **tablespoon** olive oil

7 **Oz** canned diced tomatoes with green chilies

4 **cups** fat free chicken broth

2 **cloves** garlic, minced

1 **stalk** celery, cut into 1-inch pieces

1 / 2 medium yellow onion, diced

1 / 2 medium jalapeño, seeds removed, chopped

1 / 2 medium lime, juice only

1 **teaspoon** cumin

1 / 2 **teaspoon** oregano

salt to taste

DIRECTIONS

1. Add olive oil, onion, celery, jalapeno and garlic. Sauté over medium heat until tender.

2. Add chicken breast, broth, canned tomatoes, oregano and cumin. Bring it to a boil then reduce to low heat. Cover and Simmer for 1 hour.

3. Remove the chicken from the broth. shred the meat with 2 forks then return the meat to the pot. Simmer for another 30 minutes.

4. Add lime juice and salt. Remove from heat and set aside to cool.

5. Blend the soup until smooth.

Selena's Special Tip:

- *If the puree is too thick, add extra chicken broth and blend until desired consistency is reached.*

NUTRITION FACTS (PER SERVING)

CALORIES	62	KCal
PROTEIN	9.3	g
FAT	1.6	g
CARBOHYDRATES	1.8	g
SODIUM	225	mg

FLUID AND PUREE

BUFFALO CHICKEN PUREE

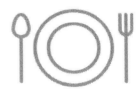

PREP TIME	COOK TIME	SERVES
5 MINUTES	10 MINUTES	10

INGREDENTS

1 **pound** boneless skinless chicken breasts

1 **tablespoon** olive oil

7 **Oz** canned diced tomatoes with green chilies

4 **cups** fat free chicken broth

2 **cloves** garlic, minced

1 **stalk** celery, cut into 1-inch pieces

1 / 2 medium yellow onion, diced

1 / 2 medium jalapeño, seeds removed, chopped

1 / 2 medium lime, juice only

1 **teaspoon** cumin

1 / 2 **teaspoon** oregano

salt to taste

DIRECTIONS

1. Cook the chicken breast in boiling water. Drain and shred into pieces. Set aside to cool.

2. Blend all ingredients until smooth.

NUTRITION FACTS (PER SERVING)

CALORIES	94	KCal
PROTEIN	10.4	g
FAT	4.5	g
CARBOHYDRATES	2.7	g
SODIUM	131	mg

FLUID AND PUREE

BEEF STEW PUREE

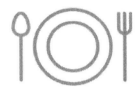

PREP TIME
10 MINUTES

COOK TIME
2 HOURS

SERVES
12

INGREDENTS

1 1/4 pounds grass-fed ground beef, 93% lean

1 tablespoon olive oil

4 Oz mushrooms, chopped

2 medium carrots, peeled and chopped

1 stalk celery, cut into 1-inch pieces

1 cup fat-free beef broth

1/2 small onion, diced

1/2 small turnip, chopped

1 tablespoon tomato paste

1 tablespoon Worcestershire Sauce

1 teaspoon oregano

salt and pepper to taste

DIRECTIONS

1. Over medium-high heat, heat the olive oil.

2. Add the ground beef. Sear for 2-3 minutes.

3. Add all vegetables. Sauté over medium heat until softened.

4. Add 1 cup of water, broth and all seasoning and stir well. Bring it to a boil and then reduce to low heat. Cover and Simmer for 1 hour and 30 minutes. Stir occasionally.

5. Set aside to cool. Blend all ingredients until smooth.

Selena's Special Tip:

- *If the puree is too thick, add extra broth and blend until desired consistency is reached.*

NUTRITION FACTS (PER SERVING)

CALORIES	94	KCal
PROTEIN	10.4	g
FAT	4.5	g
CARBOHYDRATES	2.7	g
SODIUM	131	mg

FLUID AND PUREE

CREAMY TOMATO TURKEY PUREE

PREP TIME
5 MINUTES

COOK TIME
2 HOURS

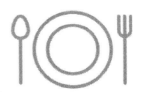

SERVES
12

INGREDENTS

1 1/2 pounds lean ground turkey

1 tablespoon olive oil

1 medium onion, diced

1 1/2 cupS vegetable broth

1/2 cup unsweetened almond milk

1 teaspoon apple cider vinegar

1 teaspoon oregano

1 teaspoon basil

salt and pepper to taste

DIRECTIONS

1. Over medium-high heat, heat the olive oil.

2. Add the turkey. Sear for 2-3 minutes.

3. Add Onion. Sauté over medium heat until softened.

4. Add broth, almond milk and all seasoning and stir well. Bring it to a boil and then reduce to low heat. Cover and Simmer for 1 hour and 30 minutes. Stir occasionally.

5. Set aside to cool. Blend all ingredients until smooth.

Selena's Special Tip:

- *If the puree is too thick, add extra broth and blend until desired consistency is reached.*

NUTRITION FACTS (PER SERVING)

CALORIES	85	KCal
PROTEIN	13.6	g
FAT	2.1	g
CARBOHYDRATES	3.2	g
SODIUM	114	mg

FLUID AND PUREE

TURKEY TETRAZZINI

PREP TIME
20 MINUTES

COOK TIME
45 MINUTES

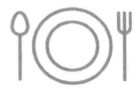

SERVES
12

INGREDENTS

1 1/2 **pounds** lean ground turkey

16 **Oz** Tofu Shirataki noodles

1 **tablespoon** olive oil

1 **cup** low fat sour cream

1 **can** mushroom soup

1/2 **cup** frozen pea

1/2 **cup** parmesan cheese, grated

salt and pepper to taste

DIRECTIONS

1. Drain Shirataki noodles. Rinse noodles under cool water. Drain and squeeze out excess water as much as possible. cut the noodles into smaller pieces.

2. Over medium-high heat, heat the olive oil.

3. Add turkey. Sear for 2-3 minutes.

4. Add frozen pea and mushroom soup. Bring it to a boil and then reduce to low heat. Simmer until the meat cooks thoroughly. Blend the mixture until smooth. Pour the mixture back to the pan.

5. Add low fat sour cream and stir well. Remove from heat and mixed with noodles.

6. Pour into a baking dish and cover the top with parmesan cheese. Bake for 20 minutes at 375 degrees.

NUTRITION FACTS (PER SERVING)

CALORIES	125	KCal
PROTEIN	14.7	g
FAT	5.2	g
CARBOHYDRATES	7.3	g
SODIUM	364	mg

FLUID AND PUREE

STEAMED TOFU WITH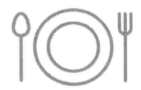

PREP TIME
5 MINUTES

COOK TIME
15 MINUTES

SERVES
4

INGREDENTS

12 Oz silken tofu

3 large egg whites, lightly beaten

1/2 teaspoon salt

DIRECTIONS

1. Mash tofu with a fork.

2. Add egg whites and mix well.

3. Divide into 4 serving dish and steamed for 10 minutes for high heat.

NUTRITION FACTS (PER SERVING)

CALORIES	138	KCal
PROTEIN	23.0	g
FAT	4.0	g
CARBOHYDRATES	5.0	g
SODIUM	356	mg

FLUID AND PUREE

GRILLED EGGPLANT YOGURT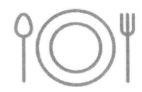

PREP TIME	COOK TIME	SERVES
5 MINUTES	30 MINUTES	4

INGREDENTS

12 Oz silken tofu

3 large egg whites, lightly beaten

1/2 teaspoon salt

DIRECTIONS

1. Broil the eggplant until skins are black and soft, turning occasionally. Remove from broiler and set aside to cool.

2. Peel Eggplant and drain. Blend the eggplant with the garlic until smooth.

3. Add salt, yogurt and cottage cheese and combine until uniform.

NUTRITION FACTS (PER SERVING)

CALORIES	96	KCal
PROTEIN	9.4	g
FAT	3.1	g
CARBOHYDRATES	8.4	g
SODIUM	427	mg

FLUID AND PUREE

CHEESY CAULIFLOWER TOFU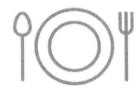

PREP TIME	COOK TIME	SERVES
5 MINUTES	20 MINUTES	12

INGREDENTS

1 large cauliflower, chopped

12 Oz silken tofu

2 cups low fat cottage cheese

1/2 cup parmesan cheese, grated

salt, pepper, garlic powder to taste

DIRECTIONS

1. Steam the cauliflower for 15 minutes or until tender.

2. Blend cauliflower, tofu, cottage cheese, parmesan cheese and seasoning until smooth.

NUTRITION FACTS (PER SERVING)

CALORIES	88	KCal
PROTEIN	10.0	g
FAT	3.1	g
CARBOHYDRATES	6.5	g
SODIUM	245	mg

FLUID AND PUREE

CLASSIC EGG SALAD

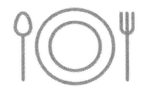

PREP TIME	COOK TIME	SERVES
5 MINUTES	5 MINUTES	4

INGREDENTS

8 hard-boiled eggs, 4 yolks and all whites, peeled

3 tablespoons low-fat mayonnaise

1 tablespoon yellow mustard

1 tablespoon lemon juice

salt and pepper to taste

DIRECTIONS

1. Blend all ingredients until smooth

NUTRITION FACTS (PER SERVING)

CALORIES	103	KCal
PROTEIN	10.0	g
FAT	5.5	g
CARBOHYDRATES	3.1	g
SODIUM	259	mg

FLUID AND PUREE

MUSHROOM CELERY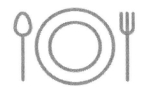

PREP TIME
10 MINUTES

COOK TIME
30 MINUTES

SERVES
6

INGREDENTS

1 **pound** mushrooms, thinly sliced

4 **strips** Celery, cut into 1-inch pieces

4 **cloves** garlic, minced

1 **tablespoon** olive oil

1 **cup** low-fat cottage cheese

1 / 2 **cup** low-fat chicken broth

salt, rosemary, sage, thyme to taste

DIRECTIONS

1. Sauté garlic, mushrooms and celery in olive oil until softened. Add spices to taste.

2. Blend the vegetables, cottage cheese and chicken broth until smooth.

NUTRITION FACTS (PER SERVING)

CALORIES	59	KCal
PROTEIN	6.8	g
FAT	0.8	g
CARBOHYDRATES	6.5	g
SODIUM	200	mg

FLUID AND PUREE

RICOTTA SPINACH CASSEROLE

PREP TIME
10 MINUTES

COOK TIME
30 MINUTES

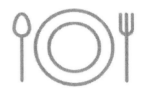

SERVES
4

INGREDENTS

10 Oz frozen spinach, thawed and drained

2 cups low-fat cottage cheese

2 large eggs, beaten

1/2 cup parmesan cheese, grated

Pinch of salt, pepper, garlic powder each

DIRECTIONS

1. Preheat the oven to 350 Degrees.

2. Blend spinach, eggs, cottage cheese and spices until smooth.

3. Pour the mixture to a baking dish and cover the top with parmesan cheese. Bake for 20-30 minutes until cheese are bubbling.

NUTRITION FACTS (PER SERVING)

CALORIES	135	KCal
PROTEIN	16.8	g
FAT	5.3	g
CARBOHYDRATES	5.2	g
SODIUM	466	mg

It's A Total Effort

As already mentioned in past chapters, gastric sleeve surgery is just a part of the journey towards your ideal weight. After you have recovered from the surgical operation, you have your work cut out for you in terms of better food choices, a more active lifestyle, and overall positive outlook that will transform your health and wellness. It's a lot of changes that you will have to get used to, but if you persevere and stick it out, it will be worth all the effort.

Take the case of Tina Tait, a sleeve gastrectomy patient at Piedmont Atlanta Hospital in Georgia. She was physically active and a regular participant in 5K runs and fundraising walks for breast cancer research, but somehow she still found it very difficult to lose weight. Before her surgical procedure, she weighed about 250 pounds.

"That was just the most helpless feeling in the world – there's nothing else I could have done that would have made me more successful," Tait said. "There's just nothing like that frustration."

Tait did not have diabetes or other conditions known as co-morbidites, so her doctor recommended that she undergo gastric sleeve surgery instead of gastric bypass or adjustable gastric band. Her physician also suggested this procedure because it would have the fastest recovery time.

Tait recalled, "After the surgery, I woke up in the hospital bed and felt like I had just had a vigorous Pilates workout. My abs were tight – I was almost unconvinced that anything had been done. I felt satisfaction for the first time in my life."

Also, Tait is quick to point out that unlike many people's misconception, weight loss surgery is not the easy way out.

"Some people say it's the easy way out and it's definitely not," she says. "[The surgery] doesn't keep you from eating things you're not supposed to eat. You still have to control what you put in your body."

Now, Tait has lost 120 pounds and weighs 130 pounds. She remains committed to the healthy lifestyle by eating right and staying active. In fact, she recently completed her first marathon.

Thank You for Reading!

Thank you very much for reading this Book and for going through the information we presented!

We realize that you have probably spent a lot of time looking elsewhere for information related to your weight loss goals, whether it is the Internet, books, magazines, newspapers, or other sources. We appreciate that you took the time to read what we have to say.

Get a BONUS gift exclusive to my readers for FREE!

- *A4-sized printable **Complete Food List Poster** for fluid and puree stages*
- *A4-sized printable Daily **Dietary Reminders Posters** for all post-surgery stages*

Scan the QR code and get yours now!

Made in the USA
Middletown, DE
30 April 2017